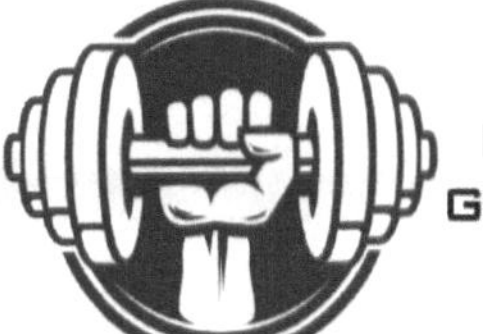

WORKOUT LOG

NAME:

GOALS:

DATE:

STATS:

WEIGHT:

EXERCISE:	SETS	REPS	WEIGHT	REST	SETS	REPS	WEIGHT	REST	SETS	REPS	WEIGHT	REST	SETS	REPS	WEIGHT	REST

CARDIO:	TIME	DIST.	INT.	PACE	TIME	DIST.	INT.	PACE	TIME	DIST.	INT.	PACE	TIME	DIST.	INT.	PACE

WORKOUT LOG

NAME:
GOALS:
DATE:
STATS:
WEIGHT:

EXERCISE:	SETS	REPS	WEIGHT	REST	SETS	REPS	WEIGHT	REST	SETS	REPS	WEIGHT	REST	SETS	REPS	WEIGHT	REST

CARDIO:	TIME	DIST.	INT.	PACE	TIME	DIST.	INT.	PACE	TIME	DIST.	INT.	PACE	TIME	DIST.	INT.	PACE

WORKOUT LOG

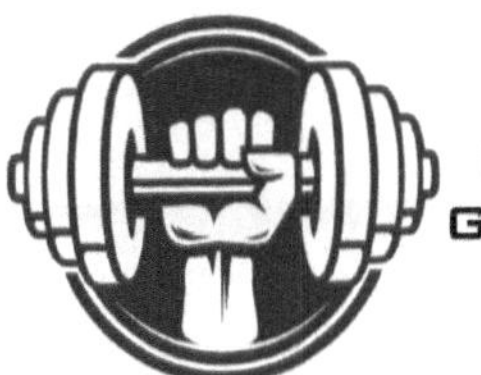

NAME:

GOALS:

DATE:

STATS:

WEIGHT:

EXERCISE:	SETS	REPS	WEIGHT	REST	SETS	REPS	WEIGHT	REST	SETS	REPS	WEIGHT	REST	SETS	REPS	WEIGHT	REST

CARDIO:	TIME	DIST.	INT.	PACE	TIME	DIST.	INT.	PACE	TIME	DIST.	INT.	PACE	TIME	DIST.	INT.	PACE

WORKOUT LOG

NAME:
GOALS:
DATE:
STATS:
WEIGHT:

EXERCISE:	SETS	REPS	WEIGHT	REST	SETS	REPS	WEIGHT	REST	SETS	REPS	WEIGHT	REST	SETS	REPS	WEIGHT	REST

CARDIO:	TIME	DIST.	INT.	PACE	TIME	DIST.	INT.	PACE	TIME	DIST.	INT.	PACE	TIME	DIST.	INT.	PACE

WORKOUT LOG

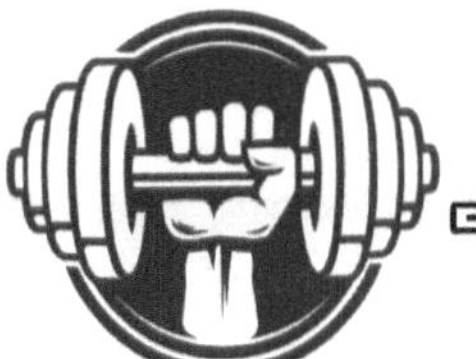

NAME:
GOALS:
DATE:
STATS:
WEIGHT:

EXERCISE:	SETS	REPS	WEIGHT	REST	SETS	REPS	WEIGHT	REST	SETS	REPS	WEIGHT	REST	SETS	REPS	WEIGHT	REST

CARDIO:	TIME	DIST.	INT.	PACE	TIME	DIST.	INT.	PACE	TIME	DIST.	INT.	PACE	TIME	DIST.	INT.	PACE

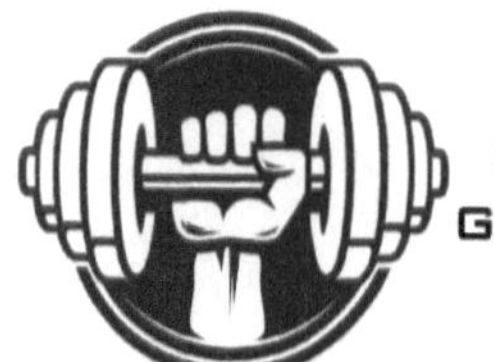

WORKOUT LOG

NAME:

GOALS:

DATE:

STATS:

WEIGHT:

EXERCISE:	SETS	REPS	WEIGHT	REST	SETS	REPS	WEIGHT	REST	SETS	REPS	WEIGHT	REST	SETS	REPS	WEIGHT	REST

CARDIO:	TIME	DIST.	INT.	PACE	TIME	DIST.	INT.	PACE	TIME	DIST.	INT.	PACE	TIME	DIST.	INT.	PACE

WORKOUT LOG

NAME:
GOALS:
DATE:
STATS:
WEIGHT:

EXERCISE:	SETS	REPS	WEIGHT	REST	SETS	REPS	WEIGHT	REST	SETS	REPS	WEIGHT	REST	SETS	REPS	WEIGHT	REST

CARDIO:	TIME	DIST.	INT.	PACE	TIME	DIST.	INT.	PACE	TIME	DIST.	INT.	PACE	TIME	DIST.	INT.	PACE

WORKOUT LOG

NAME:
GOALS:
DATE:
STATS:
WEIGHT:

EXERCISE:	SETS	REPS	WEIGHT	REST	SETS	REPS	WEIGHT	REST	SETS	REPS	WEIGHT	REST	SETS	REPS	WEIGHT	REST

CARDIO:	TIME	DIST.	INT.	PACE	TIME	DIST.	INT.	PACE	TIME	DIST.	INT.	PACE	TIME	DIST.	INT.	PACE

WORKOUT LOG

NAME:

GOALS:

DATE:

STATS:

WEIGHT:

EXERCISE:	SETS	REPS	WEIGHT	REST	SETS	REPS	WEIGHT	REST	SETS	REPS	WEIGHT	REST	SETS	REPS	WEIGHT	REST

CARDIO:	TIME	DIST.	INT.	PACE	TIME	DIST.	INT.	PACE	TIME	DIST.	INT.	PACE	TIME	DIST.	INT.	PACE

WORKOUT LOG

NAME:
GOALS:
DATE:
STATS:
WEIGHT:

EXERCISE:	SETS	REPS	WEIGHT	REST	SETS	REPS	WEIGHT	REST	SETS	REPS	WEIGHT	REST	SETS	REPS	WEIGHT	REST

CARDIO:	TIME	DIST.	INT.	PACE	TIME	DIST.	INT.	PACE	TIME	DIST.	INT.	PACE	TIME	DIST.	INT.	PACE

WORKOUT LOG

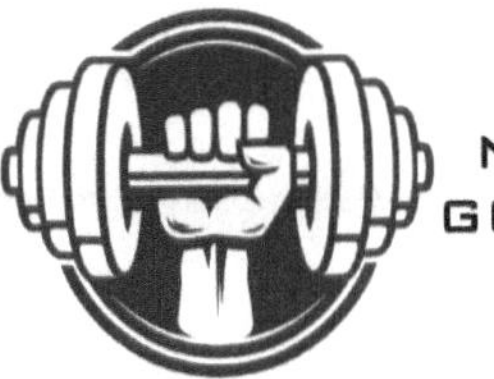

NAME:
GOALS:
DATE:
STATS:
WEIGHT:

EXERCISE:	SETS	REPS	WEIGHT	REST	SETS	REPS	WEIGHT	REST	SETS	REPS	WEIGHT	REST	SETS	REPS	WEIGHT	REST

CARDIO:	TIME	DIST.	INT.	PACE	TIME	DIST.	INT.	PACE	TIME	DIST.	INT.	PACE	TIME	DIST.	INT.	PACE

WORKOUT LOG

NAME:
GOALS:
DATE:
STATS:
WEIGHT:

EXERCISE:	SETS	REPS	WEIGHT	REST	SETS	REPS	WEIGHT	REST	SETS	REPS	WEIGHT	REST	SETS	REPS	WEIGHT	REST

CARDIO:	TIME	DIST.	INT.	PACE	TIME	DIST.	INT.	PACE	TIME	DIST.	INT.	PACE	TIME	DIST.	INT.	PACE

WORKOUT LOG

NAME:
GOALS:
DATE:
STATS:
WEIGHT:

EXERCISE:	SETS	REPS	WEIGHT	REST	SETS	REPS	WEIGHT	REST	SETS	REPS	WEIGHT	REST	SETS	REPS	WEIGHT	REST

CARDIO:	TIME	DIST.	INT.	PACE	TIME	DIST.	INT.	PACE	TIME	DIST.	INT.	PACE	TIME	DIST.	INT.	PACE

WORKOUT LOG

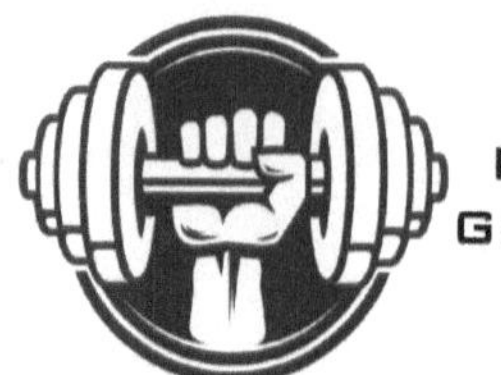

NAME:

GOALS:

DATE:

STATS:

WEIGHT:

EXERCISE:	SETS	REPS	WEIGHT	REST	SETS	REPS	WEIGHT	REST	SETS	REPS	WEIGHT	REST	SETS	REPS	WEIGHT	REST

CARDIO:	TIME	DIST.	INT.	PACE	TIME	DIST.	INT.	PACE	TIME	DIST.	INT.	PACE	TIME	DIST.	INT.	PACE

WORKOUT LOG

NAME:
GOALS:
DATE:
STATS:
WEIGHT:

EXERCISE:	SETS	REPS	WEIGHT	REST	SETS	REPS	WEIGHT	REST	SETS	REPS	WEIGHT	REST	SETS	REPS	WEIGHT	REST

CARDIO:	TIME	DIST.	INT.	PACE	TIME	DIST.	INT.	PACE	TIME	DIST.	INT.	PACE	TIME	DIST.	INT.	PACE

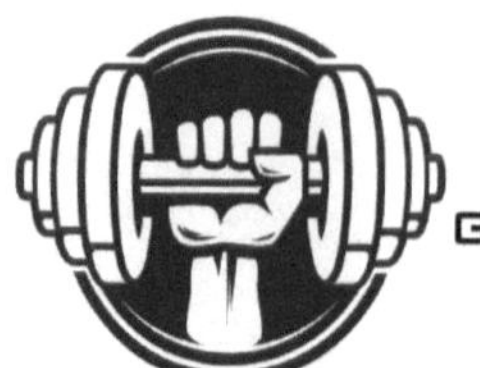

WORKOUT LOG

NAME:

GOALS:

DATE:

STATS:

WEIGHT:

EXERCISE:	SETS	REPS	WEIGHT	REST	SETS	REPS	WEIGHT	REST	SETS	REPS	WEIGHT	REST	SETS	REPS	WEIGHT	REST

CARDIO:	TIME	DIST.	INT.	PACE	TIME	DIST.	INT.	PACE	TIME	DIST.	INT.	PACE	TIME	DIST.	INT.	PACE

WORKOUT LOG

NAME:

GOALS:

DATE:

STATS:

WEIGHT:

EXERCISE:	SETS	REPS	WEIGHT	REST	SETS	REPS	WEIGHT	REST	SETS	REPS	WEIGHT	REST	SETS	REPS	WEIGHT	REST

CARDIO:	TIME	DIST.	INT.	PACE	TIME	DIST.	INT.	PACE	TIME	DIST.	INT.	PACE	TIME	DIST.	INT.	PACE

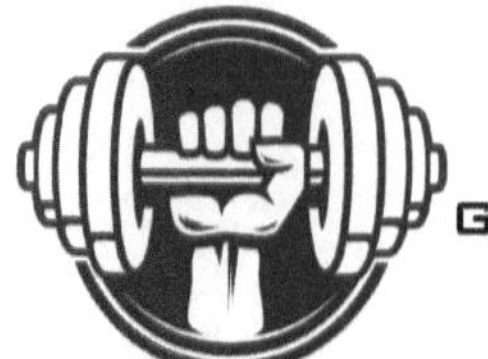

WORKOUT LOG

NAME:

GOALS:

DATE:

STATS:

WEIGHT:

EXERCISE:	SETS	REPS	WEIGHT	REST	SETS	REPS	WEIGHT	REST	SETS	REPS	WEIGHT	REST	SETS	REPS	WEIGHT	REST

CARDIO:	TIME	DIST.	INT.	PACE	TIME	DIST.	INT.	PACE	TIME	DIST.	INT.	PACE	TIME	DIST.	INT.	PACE

WORKOUT LOG

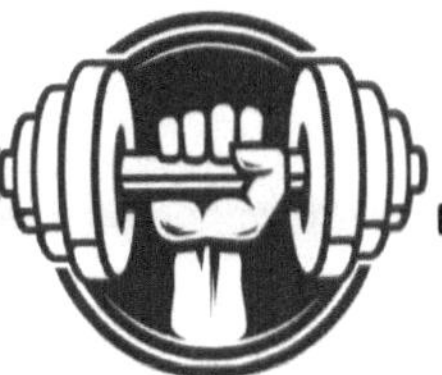

NAME: ______________________________

GOALS: ______________________________

DATE:

STATS:

WEIGHT:

EXERCISE:	SETS	REPS	WEIGHT	REST	SETS	REPS	WEIGHT	REST	SETS	REPS	WEIGHT	REST	SETS	REPS	WEIGHT	REST

CARDIO:	TIME	DIST.	INT.	PACE	TIME	DIST.	INT.	PACE	TIME	DIST.	INT.	PACE	TIME	DIST.	INT.	PACE

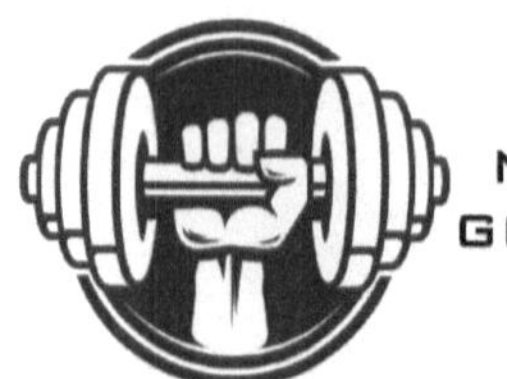

WORKOUT LOG

NAME:
GOALS:
DATE:
STATS:
WEIGHT:

EXERCISE:	SETS	REPS	WEIGHT	REST	SETS	REPS	WEIGHT	REST	SETS	REPS	WEIGHT	REST	SETS	REPS	WEIGHT	REST

CARDIO:	TIME	DIST.	INT.	PACE	TIME	DIST.	INT.	PACE	TIME	DIST.	INT.	PACE	TIME	DIST.	INT.	PACE

WORKOUT LOG

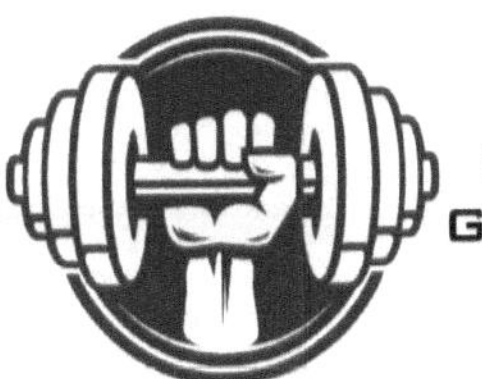

NAME:

GOALS:

DATE:

STATS:

WEIGHT:

EXERCISE:	SETS	REPS	WEIGHT	REST	SETS	REPS	WEIGHT	REST	SETS	REPS	WEIGHT	REST	SETS	REPS	WEIGHT	REST

CARDIO:	TIME	DIST.	INT.	PACE	TIME	DIST.	INT.	PACE	TIME	DIST.	INT.	PACE	TIME	DIST.	INT.	PACE

WORKOUT LOG

NAME:

GOALS:

DATE:

STATS:

WEIGHT:

EXERCISE:	SETS	REPS	WEIGHT	REST	SETS	REPS	WEIGHT	REST	SETS	REPS	WEIGHT	REST	SETS	REPS	WEIGHT	REST

CARDIO:	TIME	DIST.	INT.	PACE	TIME	DIST.	INT.	PACE	TIME	DIST.	INT.	PACE	TIME	DIST.	INT.	PACE

WORKOUT LOG

NAME:
GOALS:
DATE:
STATS:
WEIGHT:

EXERCISE:	SETS	REPS	WEIGHT	REST	SETS	REPS	WEIGHT	REST	SETS	REPS	WEIGHT	REST	SETS	REPS	WEIGHT	REST

CARDIO:	TIME	DIST.	INT.	PACE	TIME	DIST.	INT.	PACE	TIME	DIST.	INT.	PACE	TIME	DIST.	INT.	PACE

WORKOUT LOG

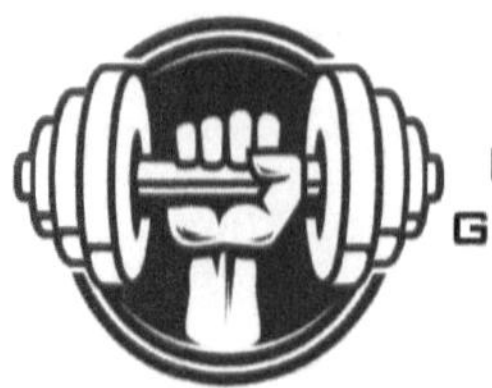

NAME:

GOALS:

DATE:

STATS:

WEIGHT:

EXERCISE:	SETS	REPS	WEIGHT	REST	SETS	REPS	WEIGHT	REST	SETS	REPS	WEIGHT	REST	SETS	REPS	WEIGHT	REST

CARDIO:	TIME	DIST.	INT.	PACE	TIME	DIST.	INT.	PACE	TIME	DIST.	INT.	PACE	TIME	DIST.	INT.	PACE

WORKOUT LOG

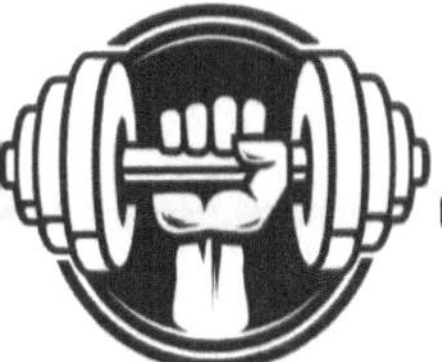

NAME:
GOALS:
DATE:
STATS:
WEIGHT:

EXERCISE:	SETS	REPS	WEIGHT	REST	SETS	REPS	WEIGHT	REST	SETS	REPS	WEIGHT	REST	SETS	REPS	WEIGHT	REST

CARDIO:	TIME	DIST.	INT.	PACE	TIME	DIST.	INT.	PACE	TIME	DIST.	INT.	PACE	TIME	DIST.	INT.	PACE

WORKOUT LOG

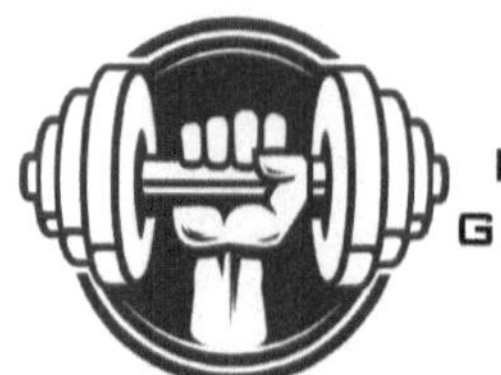

NAME:

GOALS:

DATE:

STATS:

WEIGHT:

EXERCISE:	SETS	REPS	WEIGHT	REST	SETS	REPS	WEIGHT	REST	SETS	REPS	WEIGHT	REST	SETS	REPS	WEIGHT	REST

CARDIO:	TIME	DIST.	INT.	PACE	TIME	DIST.	INT.	PACE	TIME	DIST.	INT.	PACE	TIME	DIST.	INT.	PACE

WORKOUT LOG

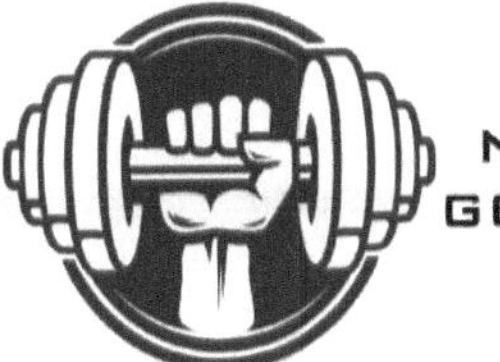

NAME:

GOALS:

DATE:

STATS:

WEIGHT:

EXERCISE:	SETS	REPS	WEIGHT	REST	SETS	REPS	WEIGHT	REST	SETS	REPS	WEIGHT	REST	SETS	REPS	WEIGHT	REST

CARDIO:	TIME	DIST.	INT.	PACE	TIME	DIST.	INT.	PACE	TIME	DIST.	INT.	PACE	TIME	DIST.	INT.	PACE

WORKOUT LOG

NAME:

GOALS:

DATE:

STATS:

WEIGHT:

EXERCISE:	SETS	REPS	WEIGHT	REST	SETS	REPS	WEIGHT	REST	SETS	REPS	WEIGHT	REST	SETS	REPS	WEIGHT	REST

CARDIO:	TIME	DIST.	INT.	PACE	TIME	DIST.	INT.	PACE	TIME	DIST.	INT.	PACE	TIME	DIST.	INT.	PACE

WORKOUT LOG

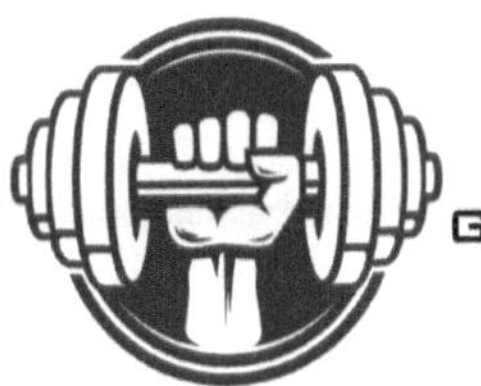

NAME:

GOALS:

DATE:

STATS:

WEIGHT:

EXERCISE:	SETS	REPS	WEIGHT	REST	SETS	REPS	WEIGHT	REST	SETS	REPS	WEIGHT	REST	SETS	REPS	WEIGHT	REST

CARDIO:	TIME	DIST.	INT.	PACE	TIME	DIST.	INT.	PACE	TIME	DIST.	INT.	PACE	TIME	DIST.	INT.	PACE

WORKOUT LOG

NAME:

GOALS:

DATE:

STATS:

WEIGHT:

EXERCISE:	SETS	REPS	WEIGHT	REST	SETS	REPS	WEIGHT	REST	SETS	REPS	WEIGHT	REST	SETS	REPS	WEIGHT	REST

CARDIO:	TIME	DIST.	INT.	PACE	TIME	DIST.	INT.	PACE	TIME	DIST.	INT.	PACE	TIME	DIST.	INT.	PACE

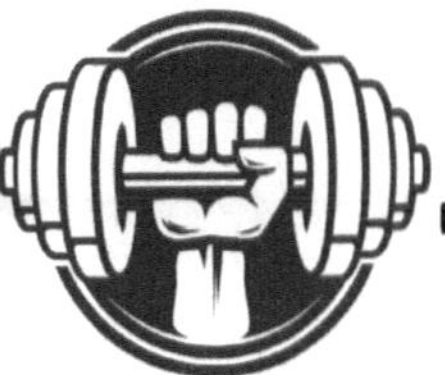

WORKOUT LOG

NAME:

GOALS:

DATE:

STATS:

WEIGHT:

EXERCISE:	SETS	REPS	WEIGHT	REST	SETS	REPS	WEIGHT	REST	SETS	REPS	WEIGHT	REST	SETS	REPS	WEIGHT	REST

CARDIO:	TIME	DIST.	INT.	PACE	TIME	DIST.	INT.	PACE	TIME	DIST.	INT.	PACE	TIME	DIST.	INT.	PACE

WORKOUT LOG

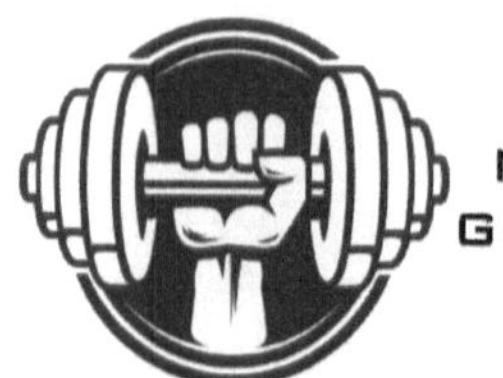

NAME:

GOALS:

DATE:

STATS:

WEIGHT:

EXERCISE:	SETS	REPS	WEIGHT	REST	SETS	REPS	WEIGHT	REST	SETS	REPS	WEIGHT	REST	SETS	REPS	WEIGHT	REST

CARDIO:	TIME	DIST.	INT.	PACE	TIME	DIST.	INT.	PACE	TIME	DIST.	INT.	PACE	TIME	DIST.	INT.	PACE

WORKOUT LOG

NAME:

GOALS:

DATE:

STATS:

WEIGHT:

EXERCISE:	SETS	REPS	WEIGHT	REST	SETS	REPS	WEIGHT	REST	SETS	REPS	WEIGHT	REST	SETS	REPS	WEIGHT	REST

CARDIO:	TIME	DIST.	INT.	PACE	TIME	DIST.	INT.	PACE	TIME	DIST.	INT.	PACE	TIME	DIST.	INT.	PACE

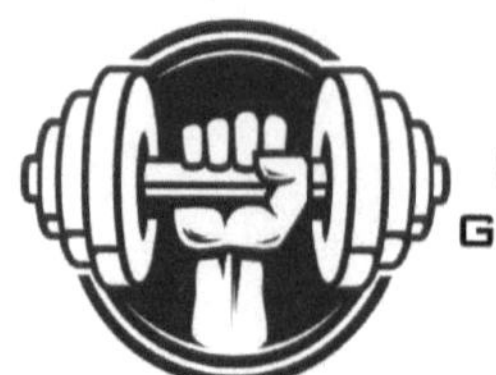

WORKOUT LOG

NAME:
GOALS:
DATE:
STATS:
WEIGHT:

EXERCISE:	SETS	REPS	WEIGHT	REST	SETS	REPS	WEIGHT	REST	SETS	REPS	WEIGHT	REST	SETS	REPS	WEIGHT	REST

CARDIO:	TIME	DIST.	INT.	PACE	TIME	DIST.	INT.	PACE	TIME	DIST.	INT.	PACE	TIME	DIST.	INT.	PACE

WORKOUT LOG

NAME:

GOALS:

DATE:

STATS:

WEIGHT:

EXERCISE:	SETS	REPS	WEIGHT	REST	SETS	REPS	WEIGHT	REST	SETS	REPS	WEIGHT	REST	SETS	REPS	WEIGHT	REST

CARDIO:	TIME	DIST.	INT.	PACE	TIME	DIST.	INT.	PACE	TIME	DIST.	INT.	PACE	TIME	DIST.	INT.	PACE

WORKOUT LOG

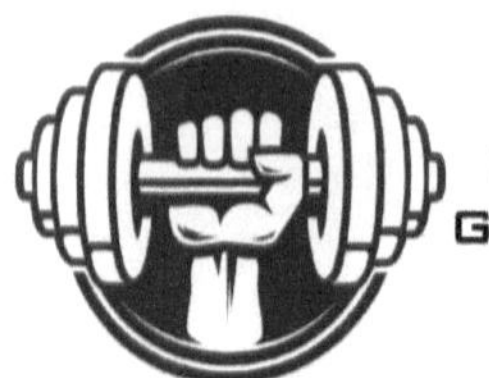

NAME:

GOALS:

DATE:

STATS:

WEIGHT:

EXERCISE:	SETS	REPS	WEIGHT	REST	SETS	REPS	WEIGHT	REST	SETS	REPS	WEIGHT	REST	SETS	REPS	WEIGHT	REST

CARDIO:	TIME	DIST.	INT.	PACE	TIME	DIST.	INT.	PACE	TIME	DIST.	INT.	PACE	TIME	DIST.	INT.	PACE

WORKOUT LOG

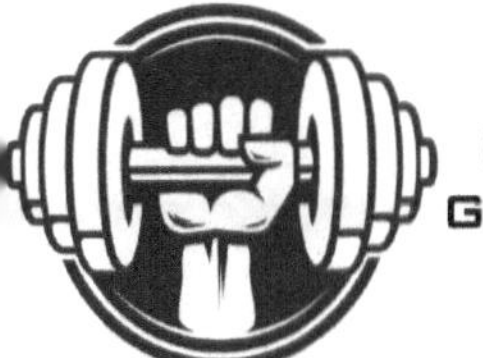

NAME:

GOALS:

DATE:

STATS:

WEIGHT:

EXERCISE:	SETS	REPS	WEIGHT	REST	SETS	REPS	WEIGHT	REST	SETS	REPS	WEIGHT	REST	SETS	REPS	WEIGHT	REST

CARDIO:	TIME	DIST.	INT.	PACE	TIME	DIST.	INT.	PACE	TIME	DIST.	INT.	PACE	TIME	DIST.	INT.	PACE

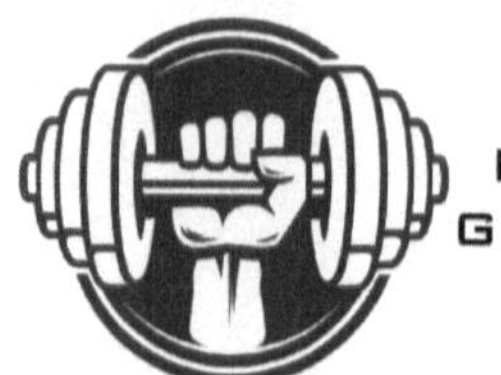

WORKOUT LOG

NAME:
GOALS:
DATE:
STATS:
WEIGHT:

EXERCISE:	SETS	REPS	WEIGHT	REST	SETS	REPS	WEIGHT	REST	SETS	REPS	WEIGHT	REST	SETS	REPS	WEIGHT	REST

CARDIO:	TIME	DIST.	INT.	PACE	TIME	DIST.	INT.	PACE	TIME	DIST.	INT.	PACE	TIME	DIST.	INT.	PACE

WORKOUT LOG

NAME:

GOALS:

DATE:

STATS:

WEIGHT:

EXERCISE:	SETS	REPS	WEIGHT	REST	SETS	REPS	WEIGHT	REST	SETS	REPS	WEIGHT	REST	SETS	REPS	WEIGHT	REST

CARDIO:	TIME	DIST.	INT.	PACE	TIME	DIST.	INT.	PACE	TIME	DIST.	INT.	PACE	TIME	DIST.	INT.	PACE

WORKOUT LOG

NAME:

GOALS:

DATE:

STATS:

WEIGHT:

EXERCISE:	SETS	REPS	WEIGHT	REST	SETS	REPS	WEIGHT	REST	SETS	REPS	WEIGHT	REST	SETS	REPS	WEIGHT	REST

CARDIO:	TIME	DIST.	INT.	PACE	TIME	DIST.	INT.	PACE	TIME	DIST.	INT.	PACE	TIME	DIST.	INT.	PACE

WORKOUT LOG

NAME:

GOALS:

DATE:

STATS:

WEIGHT:

EXERCISE:	SETS	REPS	WEIGHT	REST	SETS	REPS	WEIGHT	REST	SETS	REPS	WEIGHT	REST	SETS	REPS	WEIGHT	REST

CARDIO:	TIME	DIST.	INT.	PACE	TIME	DIST.	INT.	PACE	TIME	DIST.	INT.	PACE	TIME	DIST.	INT.	PACE

WORKOUT LOG

NAME:

GOALS:

DATE:

STATS:

WEIGHT:

EXERCISE:	SETS	REPS	WEIGHT	REST	SETS	REPS	WEIGHT	REST	SETS	REPS	WEIGHT	REST	SETS	REPS	WEIGHT	REST

CARDIO:	TIME	DIST.	INT.	PACE	TIME	DIST.	INT.	PACE	TIME	DIST.	INT.	PACE	TIME	DIST.	INT.	PACE

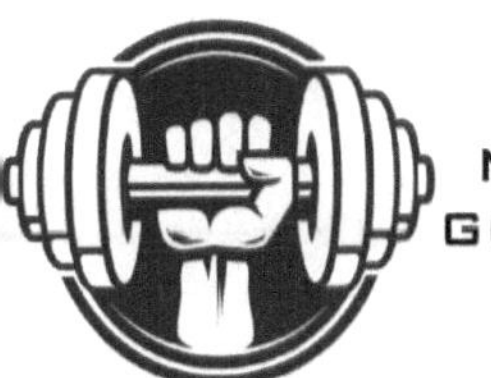

WORKOUT LOG

NAME:
GOALS:
DATE:
STATS:
WEIGHT:

EXERCISE:	SETS	REPS	WEIGHT	REST	SETS	REPS	WEIGHT	REST	SETS	REPS	WEIGHT	REST	SETS	REPS	WEIGHT	REST

CARDIO:	TIME	DIST.	INT.	PACE	TIME	DIST.	INT.	PACE	TIME	DIST.	INT.	PACE	TIME	DIST.	INT.	PACE

WORKOUT LOG

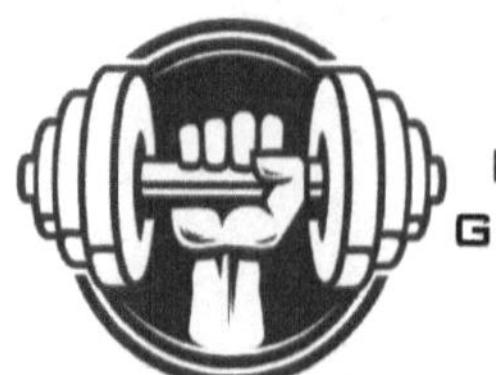

NAME:

GOALS:

DATE:

STATS:

WEIGHT:

EXERCISE:	SETS	REPS	WEIGHT	REST	SETS	REPS	WEIGHT	REST	SETS	REPS	WEIGHT	REST	SETS	REPS	WEIGHT	REST

CARDIO:	TIME	DIST.	INT.	PACE	TIME	DIST.	INT.	PACE	TIME	DIST.	INT.	PACE	TIME	DIST.	INT.	PACE

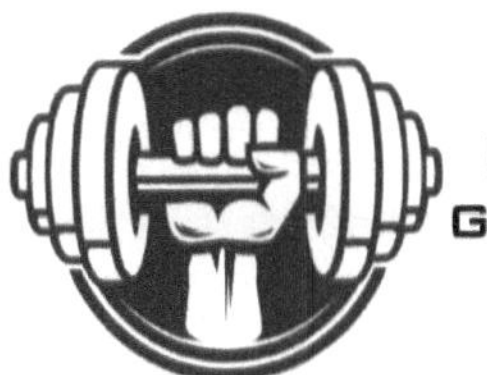

WORKOUT LOG

NAME:

GOALS:

DATE:

STATS:

WEIGHT:

EXERCISE:	SETS	REPS	WEIGHT	REST	SETS	REPS	WEIGHT	REST	SETS	REPS	WEIGHT	REST	SETS	REPS	WEIGHT	REST

CARDIO:	TIME	DIST.	INT.	PACE	TIME	DIST.	INT.	PACE	TIME	DIST.	INT.	PACE	TIME	DIST.	INT.	PACE

WORKOUT LOG

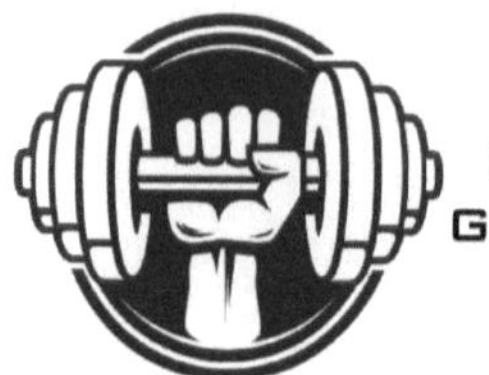

NAME:

GOALS:

DATE:

STATS:

WEIGHT:

EXERCISE:	SETS	REPS	WEIGHT	REST	SETS	REPS	WEIGHT	REST	SETS	REPS	WEIGHT	REST	SETS	REPS	WEIGHT	REST

CARDIO:	TIME	DIST.	INT.	PACE	TIME	DIST.	INT.	PACE	TIME	DIST.	INT.	PACE	TIME	DIST.	INT.	PACE

WORKOUT LOG

NAME:

GOALS:

DATE:

STATS:

WEIGHT:

EXERCISE:	SETS	REPS	WEIGHT	REST	SETS	REPS	WEIGHT	REST	SETS	REPS	WEIGHT	REST	SETS	REPS	WEIGHT	REST

CARDIO:	TIME	DIST.	INT.	PACE	TIME	DIST.	INT.	PACE	TIME	DIST.	INT.	PACE	TIME	DIST.	INT.	PACE

WORKOUT LOG

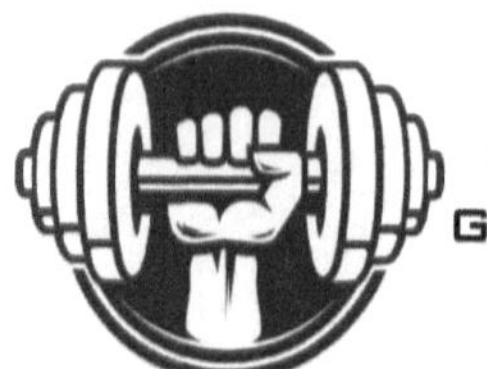

NAME:

GOALS:

DATE:

STATS:

WEIGHT:

EXERCISE:	SETS	REPS	WEIGHT	REST	SETS	REPS	WEIGHT	REST	SETS	REPS	WEIGHT	REST	SETS	REPS	WEIGHT	REST

CARDIO:	TIME	DIST.	INT.	PACE	TIME	DIST.	INT.	PACE	TIME	DIST.	INT.	PACE	TIME	DIST.	INT.	PACE

WORKOUT LOG

NAME:

GOALS:

DATE:

STATS:

WEIGHT:

EXERCISE:	SETS	REPS	WEIGHT	REST	SETS	REPS	WEIGHT	REST	SETS	REPS	WEIGHT	REST	SETS	REPS	WEIGHT	REST

CARDIO:	TIME	DIST.	INT.	PACE	TIME	DIST.	INT.	PACE	TIME	DIST.	INT.	PACE	TIME	DIST.	INT.	PACE

WORKOUT LOG

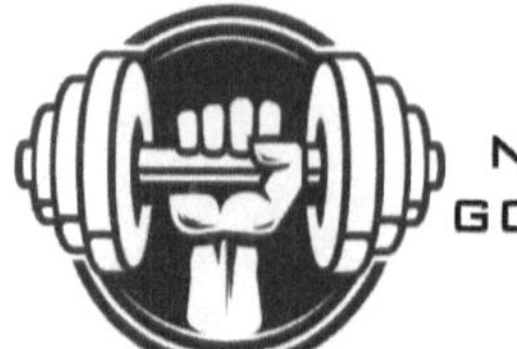

NAME:

GOALS:

DATE:

STATS:

WEIGHT:

EXERCISE:	SETS	REPS	WEIGHT	REST	SETS	REPS	WEIGHT	REST	SETS	REPS	WEIGHT	REST	SETS	REPS	WEIGHT	REST

CARDIO:	TIME	DIST.	INT.	PACE	TIME	DIST.	INT.	PACE	TIME	DIST.	INT.	PACE	TIME	DIST.	INT.	PACE

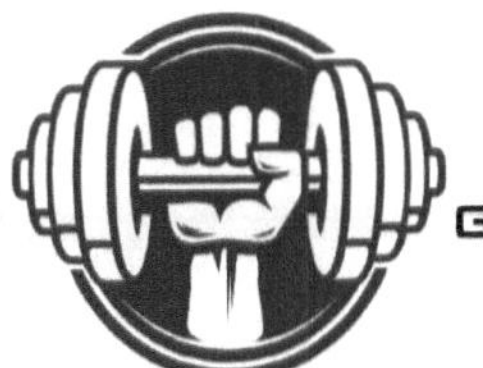

WORKOUT LOG

NAME:
GOALS:
DATE:
STATS:
WEIGHT:

EXERCISE:	SETS	REPS	WEIGHT	REST	SETS	REPS	WEIGHT	REST	SETS	REPS	WEIGHT	REST	SETS	REPS	WEIGHT	REST

CARDIO:	TIME	DIST.	INT.	PACE	TIME	DIST.	INT.	PACE	TIME	DIST.	INT.	PACE	TIME	DIST.	INT.	PACE

WORKOUT LOG

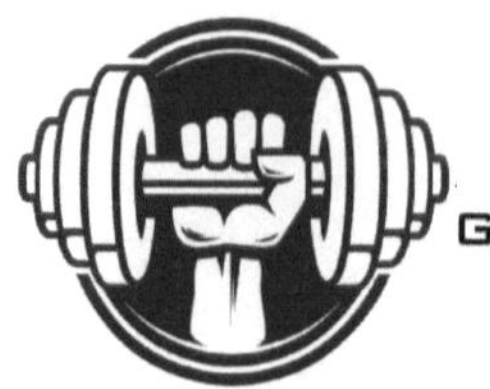

NAME:

GOALS:

DATE:

STATS:

WEIGHT:

EXERCISE:	SETS	REPS	WEIGHT	REST	SETS	REPS	WEIGHT	REST	SETS	REPS	WEIGHT	REST	SETS	REPS	WEIGHT	REST

CARDIO:	TIME	DIST.	INT.	PACE	TIME	DIST.	INT.	PACE	TIME	DIST.	INT.	PACE	TIME	DIST.	INT.	PACE

WORKOUT LOG

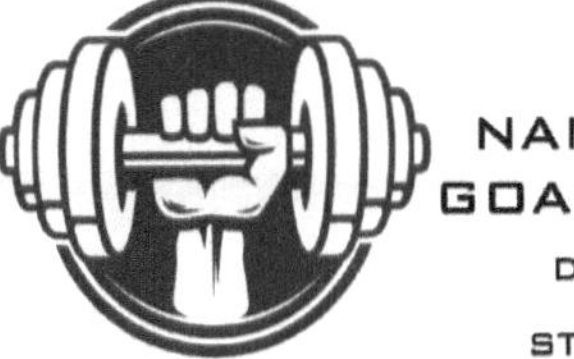

NAME:

GOALS:

DATE:

STATS:

WEIGHT:

EXERCISE:	SETS	REPS	WEIGHT	REST	SETS	REPS	WEIGHT	REST	SETS	REPS	WEIGHT	REST	SETS	REPS	WEIGHT	REST

CARDIO:	TIME	DIST.	INT.	PACE	TIME	DIST.	INT.	PACE	TIME	DIST.	INT.	PACE	TIME	DIST.	INT.	PACE

WORKOUT LOG

NAME:

GOALS:

DATE:

STATS:

WEIGHT:

EXERCISE:	SETS	REPS	WEIGHT	REST	SETS	REPS	WEIGHT	REST	SETS	REPS	WEIGHT	REST	SETS	REPS	WEIGHT	REST

CARDIO:	TIME	DIST.	INT.	PACE	TIME	DIST.	INT.	PACE	TIME	DIST.	INT.	PACE	TIME	DIST.	INT.	PACE

WORKOUT LOG

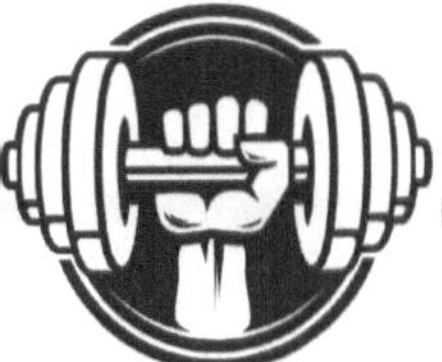

NAME:

GOALS:

DATE:

STATS:

WEIGHT:

EXERCISE:	SETS	REPS	WEIGHT	REST	SETS	REPS	WEIGHT	REST	SETS	REPS	WEIGHT	REST	SETS	REPS	WEIGHT	REST

CARDIO:	TIME	DIST.	INT.	PACE	TIME	DIST.	INT.	PACE	TIME	DIST.	INT.	PACE	TIME	DIST.	INT.	PACE

WORKOUT LOG

NAME:

GOALS:

DATE:

STATS:

WEIGHT:

EXERCISE:	SETS	REPS	WEIGHT	REST	SETS	REPS	WEIGHT	REST	SETS	REPS	WEIGHT	REST	SETS	REPS	WEIGHT	REST

CARDIO:	TIME	DIST.	INT.	PACE	TIME	DIST.	INT.	PACE	TIME	DIST.	INT.	PACE	TIME	DIST.	INT.	PACE

WORKOUT LOG

NAME:
GOALS:
DATE:
STATS:
WEIGHT:

EXERCISE:	SETS	REPS	WEIGHT	REST	SETS	REPS	WEIGHT	REST	SETS	REPS	WEIGHT	REST	SETS	REPS	WEIGHT	REST

CARDIO:	TIME	DIST.	INT.	PACE	TIME	DIST.	INT.	PACE	TIME	DIST.	INT.	PACE	TIME	DIST.	INT.	PACE

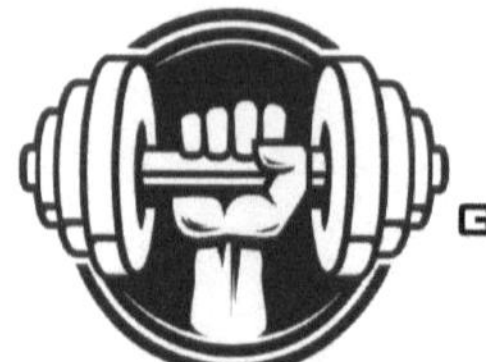

WORKOUT LOG

NAME:

GOALS:

DATE:

STATS:

WEIGHT:

EXERCISE:	SETS	REPS	WEIGHT	REST	SETS	REPS	WEIGHT	REST	SETS	REPS	WEIGHT	REST	SETS	REPS	WEIGHT	REST

CARDIO:	TIME	DIST.	INT.	PACE	TIME	DIST.	INT.	PACE	TIME	DIST.	INT.	PACE	TIME	DIST.	INT.	PACE

WORKOUT LOG

NAME:

GOALS:

DATE:

STATS:

WEIGHT:

EXERCISE:	SETS	REPS	WEIGHT	REST	SETS	REPS	WEIGHT	REST	SETS	REPS	WEIGHT	REST	SETS	REPS	WEIGHT	REST

CARDIO:	TIME	DIST.	INT.	PACE	TIME	DIST.	INT.	PACE	TIME	DIST.	INT.	PACE	TIME	DIST.	INT.	PACE

WORKOUT LOG

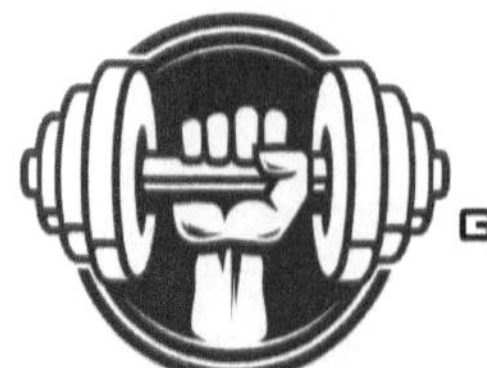

NAME:

GOALS:

DATE:

STATS:

WEIGHT:

EXERCISE:	SETS	REPS	WEIGHT	REST	SETS	REPS	WEIGHT	REST	SETS	REPS	WEIGHT	REST	SETS	REPS	WEIGHT	REST

CARDIO:	TIME	DIST.	INT.	PACE	TIME	DIST.	INT.	PACE	TIME	DIST.	INT.	PACE	TIME	DIST.	INT.	PACE

WORKOUT LOG

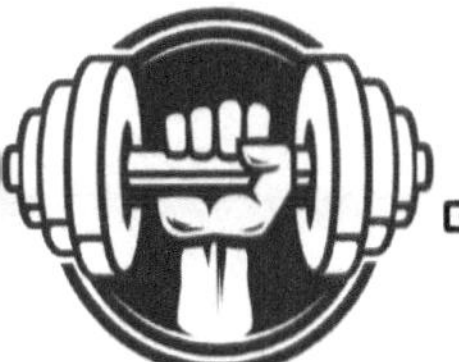

NAME:

GOALS:

DATE:

STATS:

WEIGHT:

EXERCISE:	SETS	REPS	WEIGHT	REST	SETS	REPS	WEIGHT	REST	SETS	REPS	WEIGHT	REST	SETS	REPS	WEIGHT	REST

CARDIO:	TIME	DIST.	INT.	PACE	TIME	DIST.	INT.	PACE	TIME	DIST.	INT.	PACE	TIME	DIST.	INT.	PACE

WORKOUT LOG

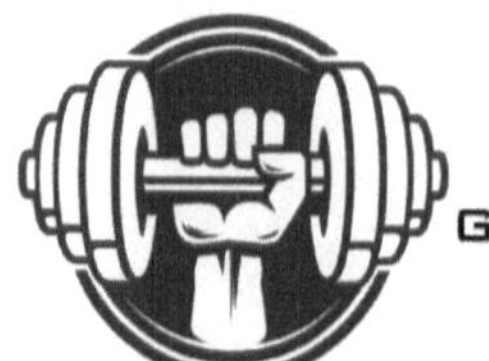

NAME:

GOALS:

DATE:

STATS:

WEIGHT:

EXERCISE:	SETS	REPS	WEIGHT	REST	SETS	REPS	WEIGHT	REST	SETS	REPS	WEIGHT	REST	SETS	REPS	WEIGHT	REST

CARDIO:	TIME	DIST.	INT.	PACE	TIME	DIST.	INT.	PACE	TIME	DIST.	INT.	PACE	TIME	DIST.	INT.	PACE

WORKOUT LOG

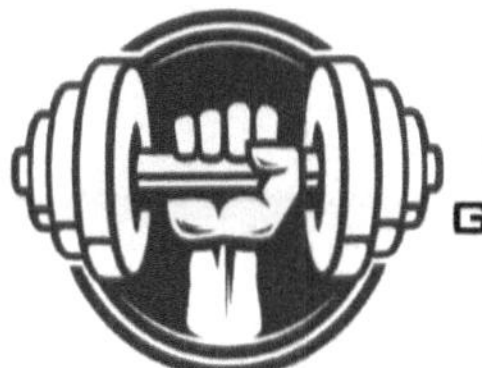

NAME:

GOALS:

DATE:

STATS:

WEIGHT:

EXERCISE:	SETS	REPS	WEIGHT	REST	SETS	REPS	WEIGHT	REST	SETS	REPS	WEIGHT	REST	SETS	REPS	WEIGHT	REST

CARDIO:	TIME	DIST.	INT.	PACE	TIME	DIST.	INT.	PACE	TIME	DIST.	INT.	PACE	TIME	DIST.	INT.	PACE

WORKOUT LOG

NAME:

GOALS:

DATE:

STATS:

WEIGHT:

EXERCISE:	SETS	REPS	WEIGHT	REST	SETS	REPS	WEIGHT	REST	SETS	REPS	WEIGHT	REST	SETS	REPS	WEIGHT	REST

CARDIO:	TIME	DIST.	INT.	PACE	TIME	DIST.	INT.	PACE	TIME	DIST.	INT.	PACE	TIME	DIST.	INT.	PACE

WORKOUT LOG

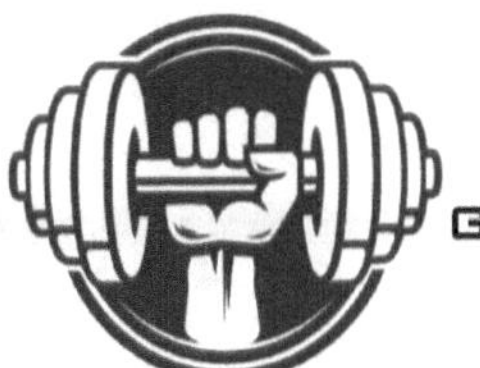

NAME:
GOALS:
DATE:
STATS:
WEIGHT:

EXERCISE:	SETS	REPS	WEIGHT	REST	SETS	REPS	WEIGHT	REST	SETS	REPS	WEIGHT	REST	SETS	REPS	WEIGHT	REST

CARDIO:	TIME	DIST.	INT.	PACE	TIME	DIST.	INT.	PACE	TIME	DIST.	INT.	PACE	TIME	DIST.	INT.	PACE

WORKOUT LOG

NAME:

GOALS:

DATE:

STATS:

WEIGHT:

EXERCISE:	SETS	REPS	WEIGHT	REST	SETS	REPS	WEIGHT	REST	SETS	REPS	WEIGHT	REST	SETS	REPS	WEIGHT	REST

CARDIO:	TIME	DIST.	INT.	PACE	TIME	DIST.	INT.	PACE	TIME	DIST.	INT.	PACE	TIME	DIST.	INT.	PACE

WORKOUT LOG

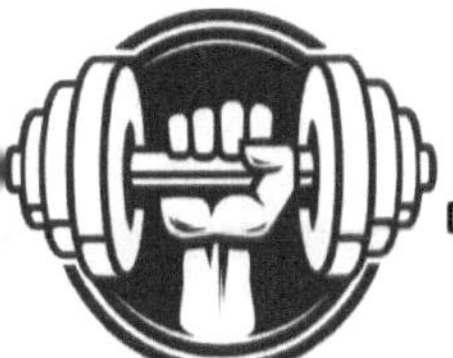

NAME:

GOALS:

DATE:

STATS:

WEIGHT:

EXERCISE:	SETS	REPS	WEIGHT	REST	SETS	REPS	WEIGHT	REST	SETS	REPS	WEIGHT	REST	SETS	REPS	WEIGHT	REST

CARDIO:	TIME	DIST.	INT.	PACE	TIME	DIST.	INT.	PACE	TIME	DIST.	INT.	PACE	TIME	DIST.	INT.	PACE

WORKOUT LOG

NAME:

GOALS:

DATE:

STATS:

WEIGHT:

EXERCISE:	SETS	REPS	WEIGHT	REST	SETS	REPS	WEIGHT	REST	SETS	REPS	WEIGHT	REST	SETS	REPS	WEIGHT	REST

CARDIO:	TIME	DIST.	INT.	PACE	TIME	DIST.	INT.	PACE	TIME	DIST.	INT.	PACE	TIME	DIST.	INT.	PACE

WORKOUT LOG

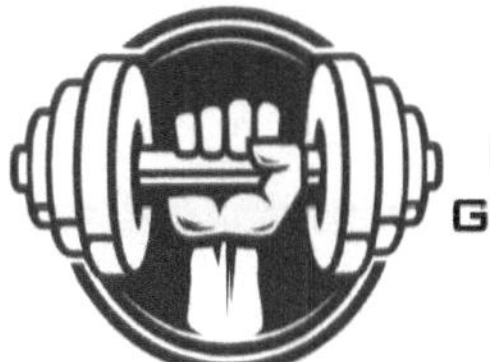

NAME:

GOALS:

DATE:

STATS:

WEIGHT:

EXERCISE:	SETS	REPS	WEIGHT	REST	SETS	REPS	WEIGHT	REST	SETS	REPS	WEIGHT	REST	SETS	REPS	WEIGHT	REST

CARDIO:	TIME	DIST.	INT.	PACE	TIME	DIST.	INT.	PACE	TIME	DIST.	INT.	PACE	TIME	DIST.	INT.	PACE

WORKOUT LOG

NAME:
GOALS:
DATE:
STATS:
WEIGHT:

EXERCISE:	SETS	REPS	WEIGHT	REST	SETS	REPS	WEIGHT	REST	SETS	REPS	WEIGHT	REST	SETS	REPS	WEIGHT	REST

CARDIO:	TIME	DIST.	INT.	PACE	TIME	DIST.	INT.	PACE	TIME	DIST.	INT.	PACE	TIME	DIST.	INT.	PACE

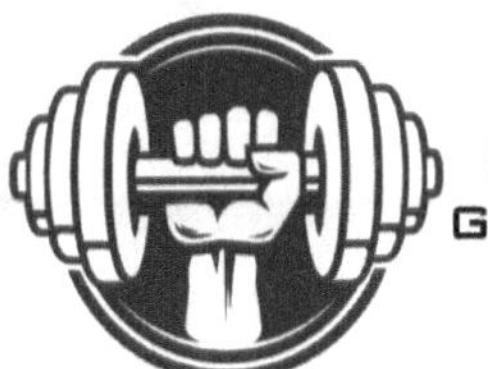

WORKOUT LOG

NAME:
GOALS:
DATE:
STATS:
WEIGHT:

EXERCISE:	SETS	REPS	WEIGHT	REST	SETS	REPS	WEIGHT	REST	SETS	REPS	WEIGHT	REST	SETS	REPS	WEIGHT	REST

CARDIO:	TIME	DIST.	INT.	PACE	TIME	DIST.	INT.	PACE	TIME	DIST.	INT.	PACE	TIME	DIST.	INT.	PACE

WORKOUT LOG

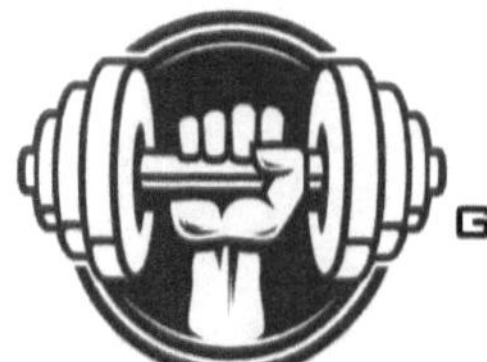

NAME:

GOALS:

DATE:

STATS:

WEIGHT:

EXERCISE:	SETS	REPS	WEIGHT	REST	SETS	REPS	WEIGHT	REST	SETS	REPS	WEIGHT	REST	SETS	REPS	WEIGHT	REST

CARDIO:	TIME	DIST.	INT.	PACE	TIME	DIST.	INT.	PACE	TIME	DIST.	INT.	PACE	TIME	DIST.	INT.	PACE

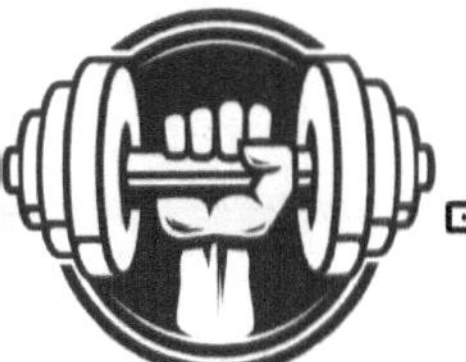

WORKOUT LOG

NAME:
GOALS:

DATE:
STATS:
WEIGHT:

EXERCISE:	SETS	REPS	WEIGHT	REST	SETS	REPS	WEIGHT	REST	SETS	REPS	WEIGHT	REST	SETS	REPS	WEIGHT	REST

CARDIO:	TIME	DIST.	INT.	PACE	TIME	DIST.	INT.	PACE	TIME	DIST.	INT.	PACE	TIME	DIST.	INT.	PACE

WORKOUT LOG

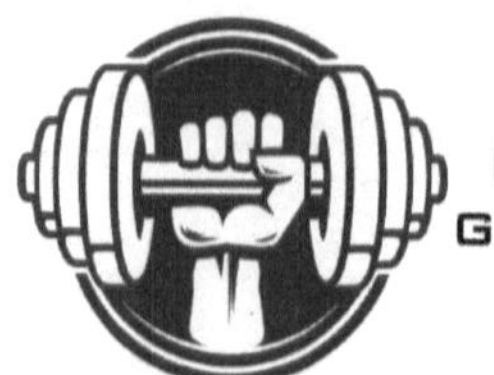

NAME:

GOALS:

DATE:

STATS:

WEIGHT:

EXERCISE:	SETS	REPS	WEIGHT	REST	SETS	REPS	WEIGHT	REST	SETS	REPS	WEIGHT	REST	SETS	REPS	WEIGHT	REST

CARDIO:	TIME	DIST.	INT.	PACE	TIME	DIST.	INT.	PACE	TIME	DIST.	INT.	PACE	TIME	DIST.	INT.	PACE

WORKOUT LOG

NAME:

GOALS:

DATE:

STATS:

WEIGHT:

EXERCISE:	SETS	REPS	WEIGHT	REST	SETS	REPS	WEIGHT	REST	SETS	REPS	WEIGHT	REST	SETS	REPS	WEIGHT	REST

CARDIO:	TIME	DIST.	INT.	PACE	TIME	DIST.	INT.	PACE	TIME	DIST.	INT.	PACE	TIME	DIST.	INT.	PACE

WORKOUT LOG

NAME:

GOALS:

DATE:

STATS:

WEIGHT:

EXERCISE:	SETS	REPS	WEIGHT	REST	SETS	REPS	WEIGHT	REST	SETS	REPS	WEIGHT	REST	SETS	REPS	WEIGHT	REST

CARDIO:	TIME	DIST.	INT.	PACE	TIME	DIST.	INT.	PACE	TIME	DIST.	INT.	PACE	TIME	DIST.	INT.	PACE

WORKOUT LOG

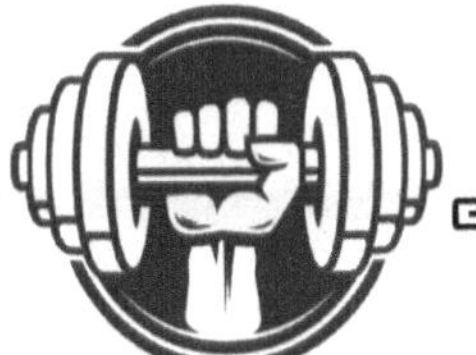

NAME:

GOALS:

DATE:

STATS:

WEIGHT:

EXERCISE:	SETS	REPS	WEIGHT	REST	SETS	REPS	WEIGHT	REST	SETS	REPS	WEIGHT	REST	SETS	REPS	WEIGHT	REST

CARDIO:	TIME	DIST.	INT.	PACE	TIME	DIST.	INT.	PACE	TIME	DIST.	INT.	PACE	TIME	DIST.	INT.	PACE

WORKOUT LOG

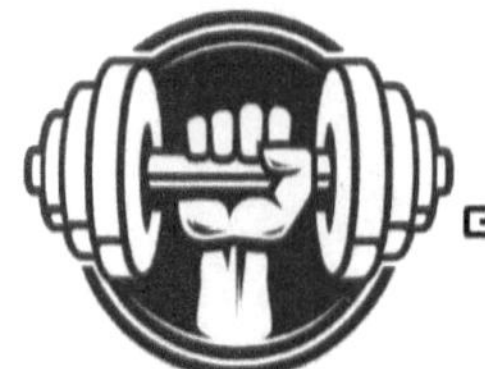

NAME:
GOALS:
DATE:
STATS:
WEIGHT:

EXERCISE:	SETS	REPS	WEIGHT	REST	SETS	REPS	WEIGHT	REST	SETS	REPS	WEIGHT	REST	SETS	REPS	WEIGHT	REST

CARDIO:	TIME	DIST.	INT.	PACE	TIME	DIST.	INT.	PACE	TIME	DIST.	INT.	PACE	TIME	DIST.	INT.	PACE

WORKOUT LOG

NAME:

GOALS:

DATE:

STATS:

WEIGHT:

EXERCISE:	SETS	REPS	WEIGHT	REST	SETS	REPS	WEIGHT	REST	SETS	REPS	WEIGHT	REST	SETS	REPS	WEIGHT	REST

CARDIO:	TIME	DIST.	INT.	PACE	TIME	DIST.	INT.	PACE	TIME	DIST.	INT.	PACE	TIME	DIST.	INT.	PACE

WORKOUT LOG

NAME:

GOALS:

DATE:

STATS:

WEIGHT:

EXERCISE:	SETS	REPS	WEIGHT	REST	SETS	REPS	WEIGHT	REST	SETS	REPS	WEIGHT	REST	SETS	REPS	WEIGHT	REST

CARDIO:	TIME	DIST.	INT.	PACE	TIME	DIST.	INT.	PACE	TIME	DIST.	INT.	PACE	TIME	DIST.	INT.	PACE

WORKOUT LOG

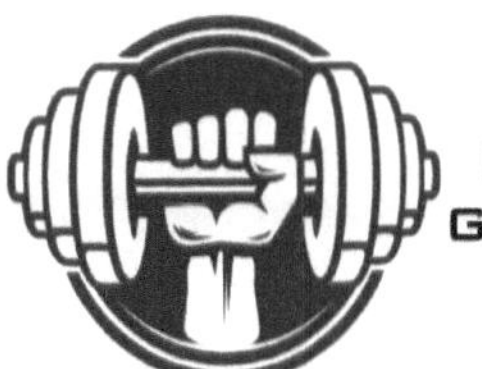

NAME:

GOALS:

DATE:

STATS:

WEIGHT:

EXERCISE:	SETS	REPS	WEIGHT	REST	SETS	REPS	WEIGHT	REST	SETS	REPS	WEIGHT	REST	SETS	REPS	WEIGHT	REST

CARDIO:	TIME	DIST.	INT.	PACE	TIME	DIST.	INT.	PACE	TIME	DIST.	INT.	PACE	TIME	DIST.	INT.	PACE

WORKOUT LOG

NAME:
GOALS:
DATE:
STATS:
WEIGHT:

EXERCISE:	SETS	REPS	WEIGHT	REST	SETS	REPS	WEIGHT	REST	SETS	REPS	WEIGHT	REST	SETS	REPS	WEIGHT	REST

CARDIO:	TIME	DIST.	INT.	PACE	TIME	DIST.	INT.	PACE	TIME	DIST.	INT.	PACE	TIME	DIST.	INT.	PACE

WORKOUT LOG

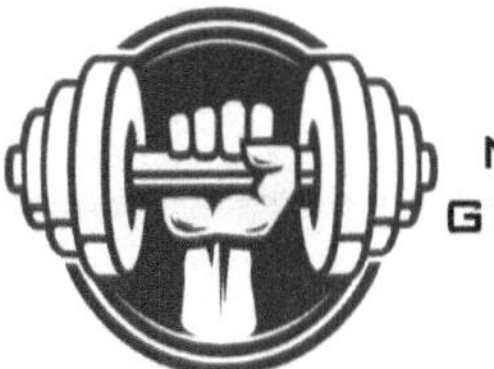

NAME:

GOALS:

DATE:

STATS:

WEIGHT:

EXERCISE:	SETS	REPS	WEIGHT	REST	SETS	REPS	WEIGHT	REST	SETS	REPS	WEIGHT	REST	SETS	REPS	WEIGHT	REST

CARDIO:	TIME	DIST.	INT.	PACE	TIME	DIST.	INT.	PACE	TIME	DIST.	INT.	PACE	TIME	DIST.	INT.	PACE

WORKOUT LOG

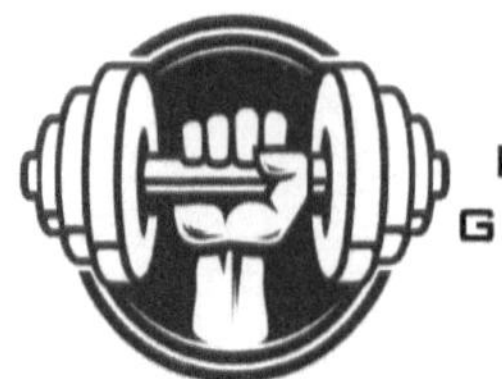

NAME:

GOALS:

DATE:

STATS:

WEIGHT:

EXERCISE:	SETS	REPS	WEIGHT	REST	SETS	REPS	WEIGHT	REST	SETS	REPS	WEIGHT	REST	SETS	REPS	WEIGHT	REST

CARDIO:	TIME	DIST.	INT.	PACE	TIME	DIST.	INT.	PACE	TIME	DIST.	INT.	PACE	TIME	DIST.	INT.	PACE

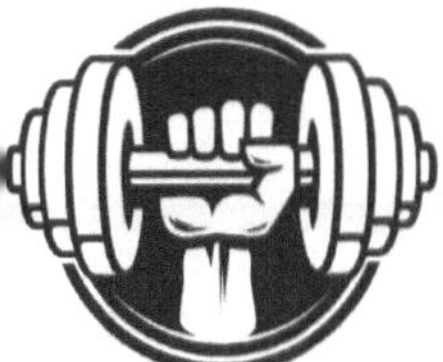

WORKOUT LOG

NAME:
GOALS:
DATE:
STATS:
WEIGHT:

EXERCISE:	SETS	REPS	WEIGHT	REST	SETS	REPS	WEIGHT	REST	SETS	REPS	WEIGHT	REST	SETS	REPS	WEIGHT	REST

CARDIO:	TIME	DIST.	INT.	PACE	TIME	DIST.	INT.	PACE	TIME	DIST.	INT.	PACE	TIME	DIST.	INT.	PACE

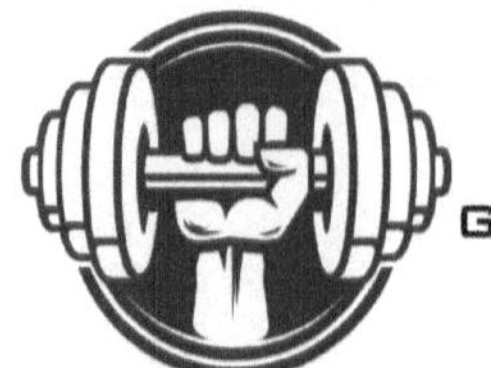

WORKOUT LOG

NAME:
GOALS:
DATE:
STATS:
WEIGHT:

EXERCISE:	SETS	REPS	WEIGHT	REST	SETS	REPS	WEIGHT	REST	SETS	REPS	WEIGHT	REST	SETS	REPS	WEIGHT	REST

CARDIO:	TIME	DIST.	INT.	PACE	TIME	DIST.	INT.	PACE	TIME	DIST.	INT.	PACE	TIME	DIST.	INT.	PACE

WORKOUT LOG

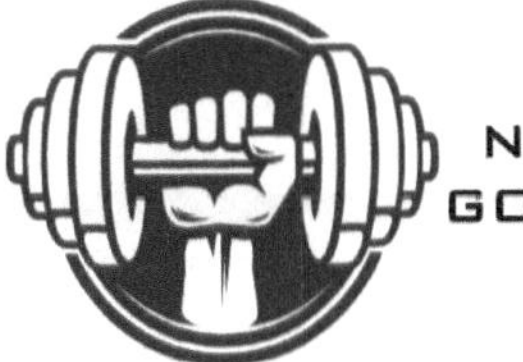

NAME:

GOALS:

DATE:

STATS:

WEIGHT:

EXERCISE:	SETS	REPS	WEIGHT	REST	SETS	REPS	WEIGHT	REST	SETS	REPS	WEIGHT	REST	SETS	REPS	WEIGHT	REST

CARDIO:	TIME	DIST.	INT.	PACE	TIME	DIST.	INT.	PACE	TIME	DIST.	INT.	PACE	TIME	DIST.	INT.	PACE

WORKOUT LOG

NAME:
GOALS:
DATE:
STATS:
WEIGHT:

EXERCISE:	SETS	REPS	WEIGHT	REST	SETS	REPS	WEIGHT	REST	SETS	REPS	WEIGHT	REST	SETS	REPS	WEIGHT	REST

CARDIO:	TIME	DIST.	INT.	PACE	TIME	DIST.	INT.	PACE	TIME	DIST.	INT.	PACE	TIME	DIST.	INT.	PACE

WORKOUT LOG

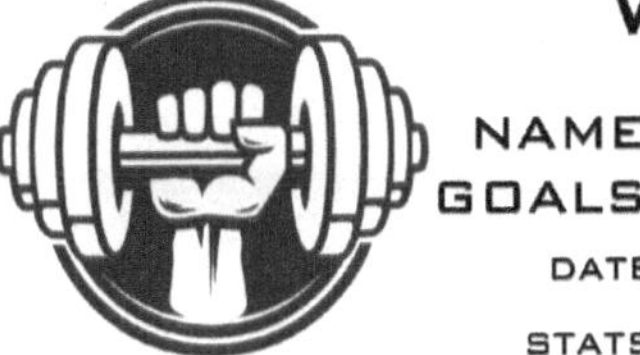

NAME:

GOALS:

DATE:

STATS:

WEIGHT:

EXERCISE:	SETS	REPS	WEIGHT	REST	SETS	REPS	WEIGHT	REST	SETS	REPS	WEIGHT	REST	SETS	REPS	WEIGHT	REST

CARDIO:	TIME	DIST.	INT.	PACE	TIME	DIST.	INT.	PACE	TIME	DIST.	INT.	PACE	TIME	DIST.	INT.	PACE

WORKOUT LOG

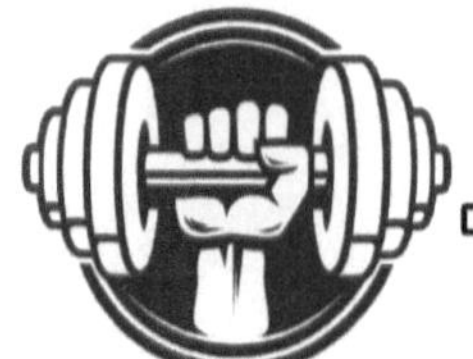

NAME: _______________________________

GOALS: _______________________________

DATE:

STATS:

WEIGHT:

EXERCISE:	SETS	REPS	WEIGHT	REST	SETS	REPS	WEIGHT	REST	SETS	REPS	WEIGHT	REST	SETS	REPS	WEIGHT	REST

CARDIO:	TIME	DIST.	INT.	PACE	TIME	DIST.	INT.	PACE	TIME	DIST.	INT.	PACE	TIME	DIST.	INT.	PACE

WORKOUT LOG

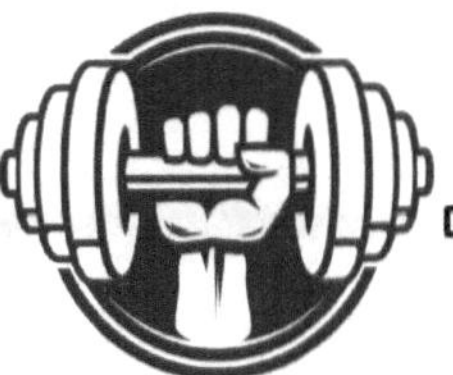

NAME:
GOALS:
DATE:
STATS:
WEIGHT:

EXERCISE:	SETS	REPS	WEIGHT	REST	SETS	REPS	WEIGHT	REST	SETS	REPS	WEIGHT	REST	SETS	REPS	WEIGHT	REST

CARDIO:	TIME	DIST.	INT.	PACE	TIME	DIST.	INT.	PACE	TIME	DIST.	INT.	PACE	TIME	DIST.	INT.	PACE

WORKOUT LOG

NAME:
GOALS:
DATE:
STATS:
WEIGHT:

EXERCISE:	SETS	REPS	WEIGHT	REST	SETS	REPS	WEIGHT	REST	SETS	REPS	WEIGHT	REST	SETS	REPS	WEIGHT	REST

CARDIO:	TIME	DIST.	INT.	PACE	TIME	DIST.	INT.	PACE	TIME	DIST.	INT.	PACE	TIME	DIST.	INT.	PACE

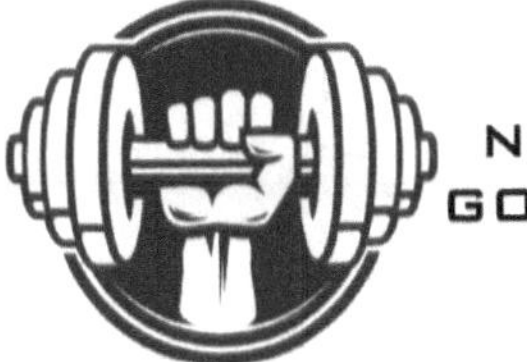

WORKOUT LOG

NAME:
GOALS:
DATE:
STATS:
WEIGHT:

EXERCISE:	SETS	REPS	WEIGHT	REST	SETS	REPS	WEIGHT	REST	SETS	REPS	WEIGHT	REST	SETS	REPS	WEIGHT	REST

CARDIO:	TIME	DIST.	INT.	PACE	TIME	DIST.	INT.	PACE	TIME	DIST.	INT.	PACE	TIME	DIST.	INT.	PACE

WORKOUT LOG

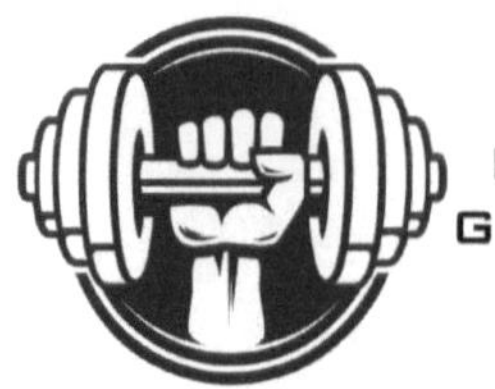

NAME:

GOALS:

DATE:

STATS:

WEIGHT:

EXERCISE:	SETS	REPS	WEIGHT	REST	SETS	REPS	WEIGHT	REST	SETS	REPS	WEIGHT	REST	SETS	REPS	WEIGHT	REST

CARDIO:	TIME	DIST.	INT.	PACE	TIME	DIST.	INT.	PACE	TIME	DIST.	INT.	PACE	TIME	DIST.	INT.	PACE

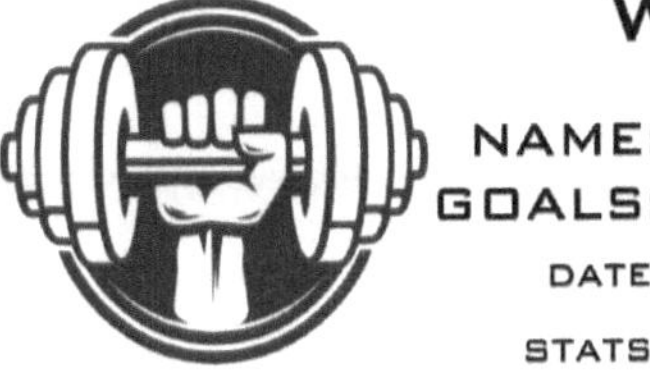

WORKOUT LOG

NAME:
GOALS:
DATE:
STATS:
WEIGHT:

EXERCISE:	SETS	REPS	WEIGHT	REST	SETS	REPS	WEIGHT	REST	SETS	REPS	WEIGHT	REST	SETS	REPS	WEIGHT	REST

CARDIO:	TIME	DIST.	INT.	PACE	TIME	DIST.	INT.	PACE	TIME	DIST.	INT.	PACE	TIME	DIST.	INT.	PACE

WORKOUT LOG

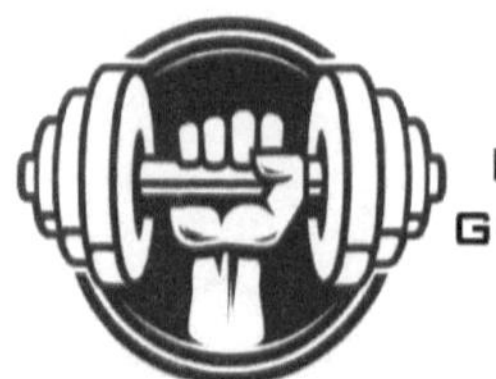

NAME:

GOALS:

DATE:

STATS:

WEIGHT:

EXERCISE:	SETS	REPS	WEIGHT	REST	SETS	REPS	WEIGHT	REST	SETS	REPS	WEIGHT	REST	SETS	REPS	WEIGHT	REST

CARDIO:	TIME	DIST.	INT.	PACE	TIME	DIST.	INT.	PACE	TIME	DIST.	INT.	PACE	TIME	DIST.	INT.	PACE

WORKOUT LOG

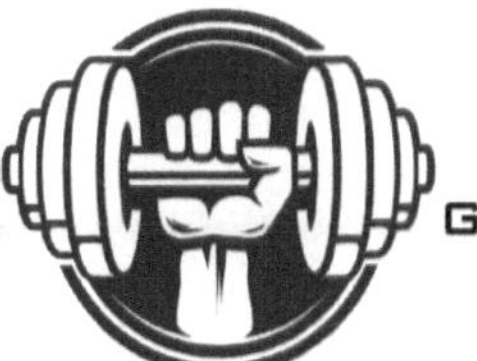

NAME:

GOALS:

DATE:

STATS:

WEIGHT:

EXERCISE:	SETS	REPS	WEIGHT	REST	SETS	REPS	WEIGHT	REST	SETS	REPS	WEIGHT	REST	SETS	REPS	WEIGHT	REST

CARDIO:	TIME	DIST.	INT.	PACE	TIME	DIST.	INT.	PACE	TIME	DIST.	INT.	PACE	TIME	DIST.	INT.	PACE

WORKOUT LOG

NAME:
GOALS:
DATE:
STATS:
WEIGHT:

EXERCISE:	SETS	REPS	WEIGHT	REST	SETS	REPS	WEIGHT	REST	SETS	REPS	WEIGHT	REST	SETS	REPS	WEIGHT	REST

CARDIO:	TIME	DIST.	INT.	PACE	TIME	DIST.	INT.	PACE	TIME	DIST.	INT.	PACE	TIME	DIST.	INT.	PACE

WORKOUT LOG

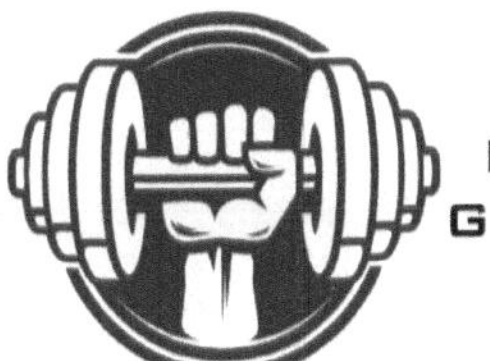

NAME:

GOALS:

DATE:

STATS:

WEIGHT:

EXERCISE:	SETS	REPS	WEIGHT	REST	SETS	REPS	WEIGHT	REST	SETS	REPS	WEIGHT	REST	SETS	REPS	WEIGHT	REST

CARDIO:	TIME	DIST.	INT.	PACE	TIME	DIST.	INT.	PACE	TIME	DIST.	INT.	PACE	TIME	DIST.	INT.	PACE

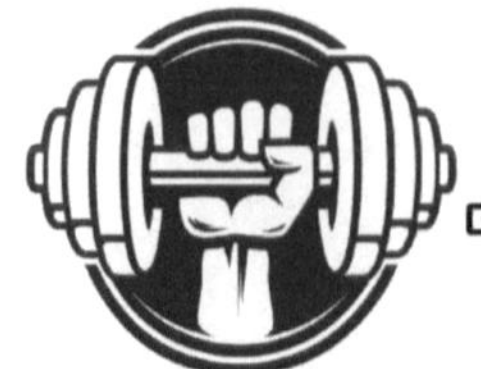

WORKOUT LOG

NAME: _______________

GOALS: _______________

DATE: ___ ___ ___ ___

STATS: ___ ___ ___ ___

WEIGHT: ___ ___ ___ ___

EXERCISE:	SETS	REPS	WEIGHT	REST	SETS	REPS	WEIGHT	REST	SETS	REPS	WEIGHT	REST	SETS	REPS	WEIGHT	REST

CARDIO:	TIME	DIST.	INT.	PACE	TIME	DIST.	INT.	PACE	TIME	DIST.	INT.	PACE	TIME	DIST.	INT.	PACE

WORKOUT LOG

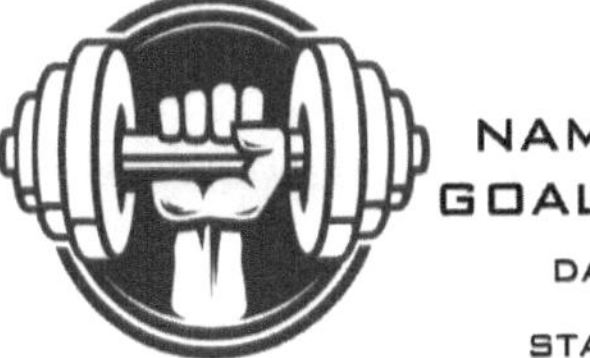

NAME:

GOALS:

DATE:

STATS:

WEIGHT:

EXERCISE:	SETS	REPS	WEIGHT	REST	SETS	REPS	WEIGHT	REST	SETS	REPS	WEIGHT	REST	SETS	REPS	WEIGHT	REST

CARDIO:	TIME	DIST.	INT.	PACE	TIME	DIST.	INT.	PACE	TIME	DIST.	INT.	PACE	TIME	DIST.	INT.	PACE

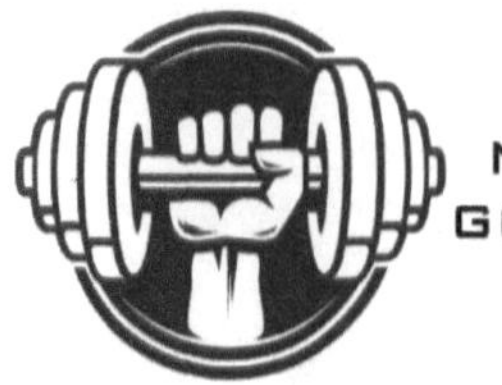

WORKOUT LOG

NAME:

GOALS:

DATE:

STATS:

WEIGHT:

EXERCISE:	SETS	REPS	WEIGHT	REST	SETS	REPS	WEIGHT	REST	SETS	REPS	WEIGHT	REST	SETS	REPS	WEIGHT	REST

CARDIO:	TIME	DIST.	INT.	PACE	TIME	DIST.	INT.	PACE	TIME	DIST.	INT.	PACE	TIME	DIST.	INT.	PACE

WORKOUT LOG

NAME:

GOALS:

DATE:

STATS:

WEIGHT:

EXERCISE:	SETS	REPS	WEIGHT	REST	SETS	REPS	WEIGHT	REST	SETS	REPS	WEIGHT	REST	SETS	REPS	WEIGHT	REST

CARDIO:	TIME	DIST.	INT.	PACE	TIME	DIST.	INT.	PACE	TIME	DIST.	INT.	PACE	TIME	DIST.	INT.	PACE

WORKOUT LOG

NAME:

GOALS:

DATE:

STATS:

WEIGHT:

EXERCISE:	SETS	REPS	WEIGHT	REST	SETS	REPS	WEIGHT	REST	SETS	REPS	WEIGHT	REST	SETS	REPS	WEIGHT	REST

CARDIO:	TIME	DIST.	INT.	PACE	TIME	DIST.	INT.	PACE	TIME	DIST.	INT.	PACE	TIME	DIST.	INT.	PACE

WORKOUT LOG

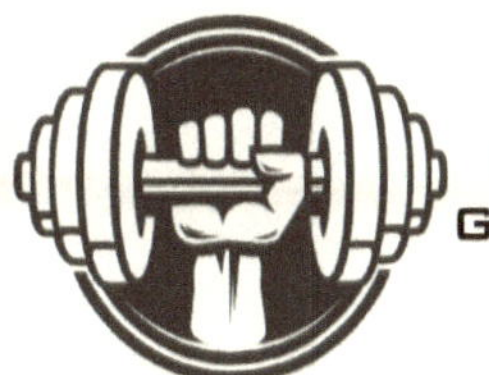

NAME:

GOALS:

DATE:

STATS:

WEIGHT:

EXERCISE:	SETS	REPS	WEIGHT	REST	SETS	REPS	WEIGHT	REST	SETS	REPS	WEIGHT	REST	SETS	REPS	WEIGHT	REST

CARDIO:	TIME	DIST.	INT.	PACE	TIME	DIST.	INT.	PACE	TIME	DIST.	INT.	PACE	TIME	DIST.	INT.	PACE

WORKOUT LOG

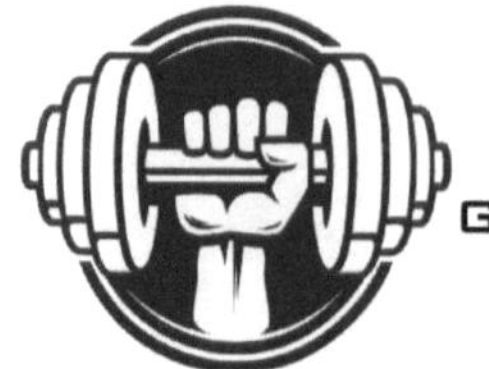

NAME:

GOALS:

DATE:

STATS:

WEIGHT:

EXERCISE:	SETS	REPS	WEIGHT	REST	SETS	REPS	WEIGHT	REST	SETS	REPS	WEIGHT	REST	SETS	REPS	WEIGHT	REST

CARDIO:	TIME	DIST.	INT.	PACE	TIME	DIST.	INT.	PACE	TIME	DIST.	INT.	PACE	TIME	DIST.	INT.	PACE

WORKOUT LOG

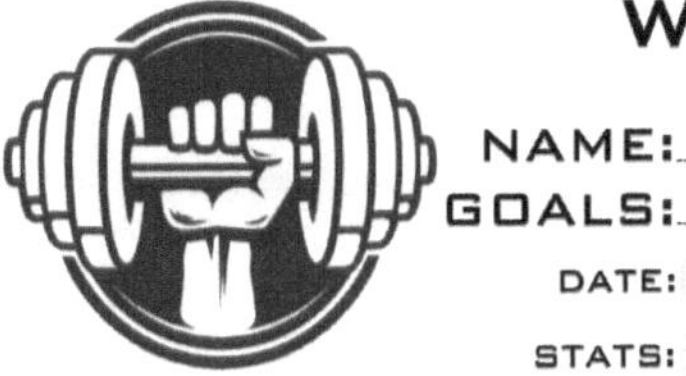

NAME:

GOALS:

DATE:

STATS:

WEIGHT:

EXERCISE:	SETS	REPS	WEIGHT	REST	SETS	REPS	WEIGHT	REST	SETS	REPS	WEIGHT	REST	SETS	REPS	WEIGHT	REST

CARDIO:	TIME	DIST.	INT.	PACE	TIME	DIST.	INT.	PACE	TIME	DIST.	INT.	PACE	TIME	DIST.	INT.	PACE

WORKOUT LOG

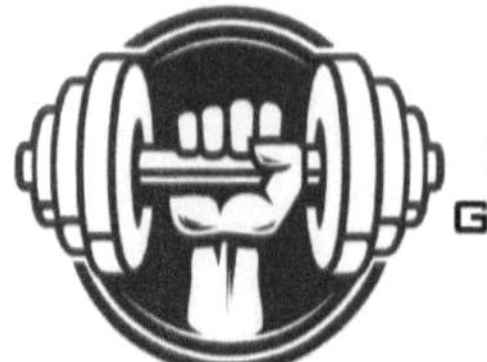

NAME:

GOALS:

DATE:			
STATS:			
WEIGHT:			

EXERCISE:	SETS	REPS	WEIGHT	REST	SETS	REPS	WEIGHT	REST	SETS	REPS	WEIGHT	REST	SETS	REPS	WEIGHT	REST

CARDIO:	TIME	DIST.	INT.	PACE	TIME	DIST.	INT.	PACE	TIME	DIST.	INT.	PACE	TIME	DIST.	INT.	PACE

WORKOUT LOG

NAME:

GOALS:

DATE:

STATS:

WEIGHT:

EXERCISE:	SETS	REPS	WEIGHT	REST	SETS	REPS	WEIGHT	REST	SETS	REPS	WEIGHT	REST	SETS	REPS	WEIGHT	REST

CARDIO:	TIME	DIST.	INT.	PACE	TIME	DIST.	INT.	PACE	TIME	DIST.	INT.	PACE	TIME	DIST.	INT.	PACE

WORKOUT LOG

NAME: ___________________________

GOALS: ___________________________

DATE:

STATS:

WEIGHT:

EXERCISE:	SETS	REPS	WEIGHT	REST	SETS	REPS	WEIGHT	REST	SETS	REPS	WEIGHT	REST	SETS	REPS	WEIGHT	REST

CARDIO:	TIME	DIST.	INT.	PACE	TIME	DIST.	INT.	PACE	TIME	DIST.	INT.	PACE	TIME	DIST.	INT.	PACE

WORKOUT LOG

NAME:_____________________________

GOALS:_____________________________

DATE:

STATS:

WEIGHT:

EXERCISE:	SETS	REPS	WEIGHT	REST	SETS	REPS	WEIGHT	REST	SETS	REPS	WEIGHT	REST	SETS	REPS	WEIGHT	REST

CARDIO:	TIME	DIST.	INT.	PACE	TIME	DIST.	INT.	PACE	TIME	DIST.	INT.	PACE	TIME	DIST.	INT.	PACE

WORKOUT LOG

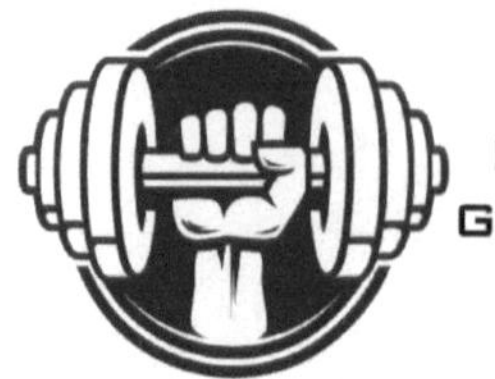

NAME:

GOALS:

DATE:

STATS:

WEIGHT:

EXERCISE:	SETS	REPS	WEIGHT	REST	SETS	REPS	WEIGHT	REST	SETS	REPS	WEIGHT	REST	SETS	REPS	WEIGHT	REST

CARDIO:	TIME	DIST.	INT.	PACE	TIME	DIST.	INT.	PACE	TIME	DIST.	INT.	PACE	TIME	DIST.	INT.	PACE

WORKOUT LOG

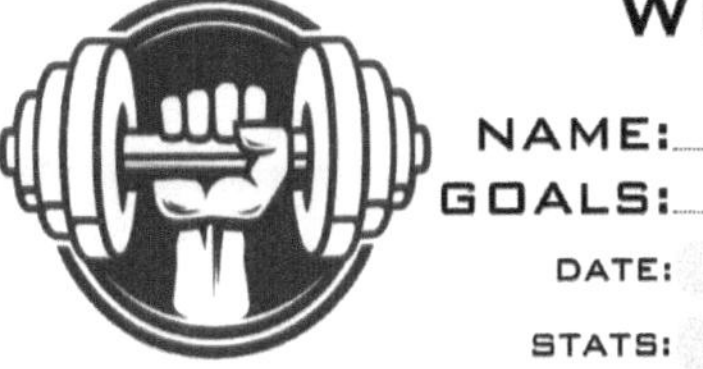

NAME:

GOALS:

DATE:

STATS:

WEIGHT:

EXERCISE:	SETS	REPS	WEIGHT	REST	SETS	REPS	WEIGHT	REST	SETS	REPS	WEIGHT	REST	SETS	REPS	WEIGHT	REST

CARDIO:	TIME	DIST.	INT.	PACE	TIME	DIST.	INT.	PACE	TIME	DIST.	INT.	PACE	TIME	DIST.	INT.	PACE

WORKOUT LOG

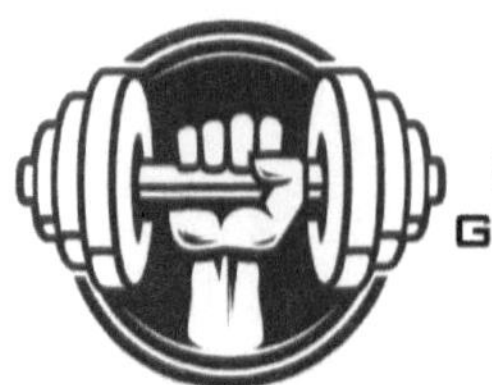

NAME:

GOALS:

DATE:

STATS:

WEIGHT:

EXERCISE:	SETS	REPS	WEIGHT	REST	SETS	REPS	WEIGHT	REST	SETS	REPS	WEIGHT	REST	SETS	REPS	WEIGHT	REST

CARDIO:	TIME	DIST.	INT.	PACE	TIME	DIST.	INT.	PACE	TIME	DIST.	INT.	PACE	TIME	DIST.	INT.	PACE

WORKOUT LOG

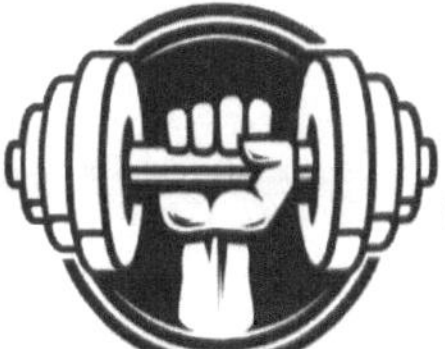

NAME:

GOALS:

DATE:

STATS:

WEIGHT:

EXERCISE:	SETS	REPS	WEIGHT	REST	SETS	REPS	WEIGHT	REST	SETS	REPS	WEIGHT	REST	SETS	REPS	WEIGHT	REST

CARDIO:	TIME	DIST.	INT.	PACE	TIME	DIST.	INT.	PACE	TIME	DIST.	INT.	PACE	TIME	DIST.	INT.	PACE

WORKOUT LOG

NAME:

GOALS:

DATE:

STATS:

WEIGHT:

EXERCISE:	SETS	REPS	WEIGHT	REST	SETS	REPS	WEIGHT	REST	SETS	REPS	WEIGHT	REST	SETS	REPS	WEIGHT	REST

CARDIO:	TIME	DIST.	INT.	PACE	TIME	DIST.	INT.	PACE	TIME	DIST.	INT.	PACE	TIME	DIST.	INT.	PACE

WORKOUT LOG

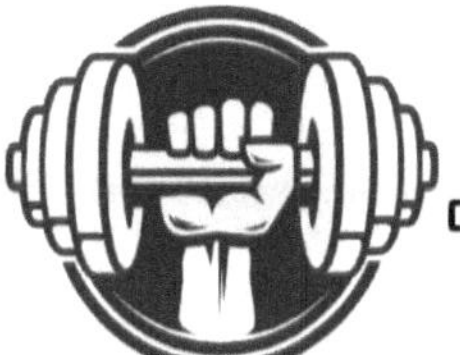

NAME:

GOALS:

DATE:

STATS:

WEIGHT:

EXERCISE:	SETS	REPS	WEIGHT	REST	SETS	REPS	WEIGHT	REST	SETS	REPS	WEIGHT	REST	SETS	REPS	WEIGHT	REST

CARDIO:	TIME	DIST.	INT.	PACE	TIME	DIST.	INT.	PACE	TIME	DIST.	INT.	PACE	TIME	DIST.	INT.	PACE

WORKOUT LOG

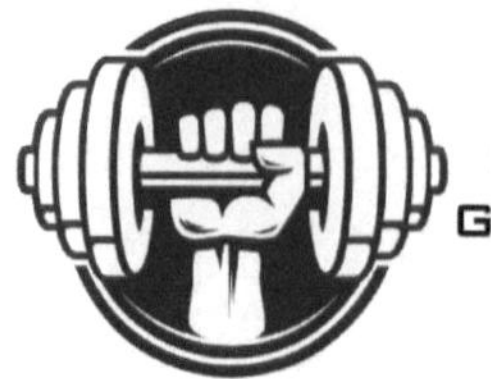

NAME:

GOALS:

DATE:

STATS:

WEIGHT:

EXERCISE:	SETS	REPS	WEIGHT	REST	SETS	REPS	WEIGHT	REST	SETS	REPS	WEIGHT	REST	SETS	REPS	WEIGHT	REST

CARDIO:	TIME	DIST.	INT.	PACE	TIME	DIST.	INT.	PACE	TIME	DIST.	INT.	PACE	TIME	DIST.	INT.	PACE

WORKOUT LOG

NAME:
GOALS:
DATE:
STATS:
WEIGHT:

EXERCISE:	SETS	REPS	WEIGHT	REST	SETS	REPS	WEIGHT	REST	SETS	REPS	WEIGHT	REST	SETS	REPS	WEIGHT	REST

CARDIO:	TIME	DIST.	INT.	PACE	TIME	DIST.	INT.	PACE	TIME	DIST.	INT.	PACE	TIME	DIST.	INT.	PACE

WORKOUT LOG

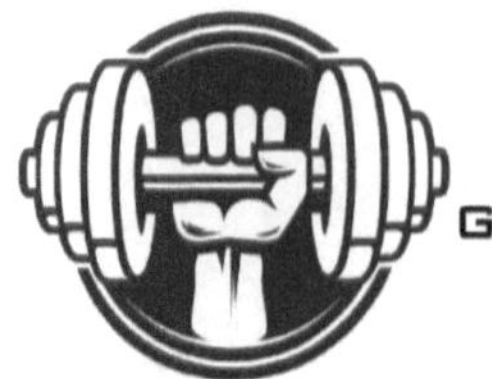

NAME:

GOALS:

DATE:

STATS:

WEIGHT:

EXERCISE:	SETS	REPS	WEIGHT	REST	SETS	REPS	WEIGHT	REST	SETS	REPS	WEIGHT	REST	SETS	REPS	WEIGHT	REST

CARDIO:	TIME	DIST.	INT.	PACE	TIME	DIST.	INT.	PACE	TIME	DIST.	INT.	PACE	TIME	DIST.	INT.	PACE